Distribution, publication, and copying in any form are prohibited and subject to damages.

TEN HYPNOSES

Copying, publishing, and sharing with third parties are only permitted with the written consent of the author. Please observe the notes on copyright and usage.

Distribution, publication, and copying in any form are prohibited and subject to damages.

Copying, publishing, and sharing with third parties are only permitted with the written consent of the author. Please observe the notes on copyright and usage.

Distribution, publication, and copying in any form are prohibited and subject to damages.

Ingo Michael Simon

TEN HYPNOSES

49

BULIMIA

Copying, publishing, and sharing with third parties are only permitted with the written consent of the author. Please observe the notes on copyright and usage.

Distribution, publication, and copying in any form are prohibited and subject to damages.

© 2024 Ingo Michael Simon
All rights reserved.
Independently published
www.ingosimon.com

Important Notes for Urgent Attention:

The contents of this book are based on the practical experiences of the author with hypnosis applications and psychotherapy in a trance state. Although the author has strived for the utmost care, errors or misunderstandings in the presentation cannot be completely excluded. Therapeutic work with people and the application of hypnosis are solely the responsibility of the hypnotist. It cannot be ruled out that parts of this book may be misunderstood or that the application of a presented procedure may cause an undesirable reaction in the client. The author also assumes no co-responsibility if work with a client is carried out with reference to the statements in this book.

The Author:

Ingo Michael Simon studied psychology and education and is a hypnotherapist with practices in southwestern Germany and Switzerland. With the help of hypnosis-supported psychotherapy, he primarily treats people with persistent psychological conditions. His practice focuses on anxiety disorders, pathological compulsions, and psychosomatic illnesses. His therapeutic offerings mainly include classical and modern hypnosis applications and the dreamland therapy he developed himself.

Copying, publishing, and sharing with third parties are only permitted with the written consent of the author. Please observe the notes on copyright and usage.

Distribution, publication, and copying in any form are prohibited and subject to damages.

INTRODUCTION	6
COPYRIGHT AND USAGE	8
HYPNOSIS 1	10
HYPNOSIS 2	15
HYPNOSIS 3	23
HYPNOSIS 4	29
HYPNOSIS 5	35
HYPNOSIS 6	41
HYPNOSIS 7	45
HYPNOSIS 8	52
HYPNOSIS 9	60
HYPNOSIS 10	67
ALL TITLES IN THE SERIES	73

Copying, publishing, and sharing with third parties are only permitted with the written consent of the author. Please observe the notes on copyright and usage.

Distribution, publication, and copying in any form are prohibited and subject to damages.

Introduction

The series "Ten Hypnoses" is very well known in Germany, Austria, and Switzerland as a collection of texts for therapeutic work and is used by numerous psychotherapeutic practices, doctors, therapists, coaches, and other helping professionals. I am pleased to now be able to offer these texts in other countries as well.

Most therapists have their own methods for inducing and deepening trance as well as for exiting trance. Therefore, I have focused on the main part of the hypnosis. The texts in this book can be integrated as the main part into any hypnosis process. The texts in this collection use various hypnosis techniques. I will not explain these in detail, as I assume that users have the appropriate training. It is also not necessary to understand the exact structure or functioning of the different parts. The texts can simply be read aloud, and they will have their effect.

Decide for yourself which text best suits your client or patient at any given time. You can also combine passages from different texts. It is not about using all ten hypnoses in sequence. It is a selection of possibilities.

Copying, publishing, and sharing with third parties are only permitted with the written consent of the author. Please observe the notes on copyright and usage.

I want to emphasize that books cannot replace therapy. Psychotherapy or other therapeutic treatments involve much more. A careful diagnosis is the necessary basis for deciding on the use of methods, including whether hypnosis or one of my texts should be used. Even in this case, preparatory discussions, follow-up discussions during the session, and of course, a therapeutic concept for the sequence of sessions and the content approaches are essential parts of therapy. This cannot and should not be achieved with a collection of texts.

In any case, I wish you much success in your work and I am pleased if my text templates can contribute in a small way.

Ingo Michael Simon

Distribution, publication, and copying in any form are prohibited and subject to damages.

Copyright and Usage

Copying, publishing, and sharing with third parties is prohibited and only permitted with the written consent of the author. Please observe the following copyright and usage guidelines.

This work has been carefully crafted and created to the best of the author's knowledge and personal experience. It comprises text templates and application guidelines for professional hypnosis sessions. The author is a licensed psychotherapist with extensive experience in psychotherapy, coaching, and personal training using hypnotic techniques and methods. Nevertheless, the author and the publisher assume no liability for the accuracy of information, instructions, and advice, nor for any typographical errors. The author and publisher accept no responsibility or liability for the application of these texts and recommendations with clients or patients, nor for any potential consequences or unexpected reactions. It is expressly noted that the application of therapeutic and advisory techniques and formulations lies solely and entirely within the responsibility of the practitioner. This also applies to adherence to the

Copying, publishing, and sharing with third parties are only permitted with the written consent of the author. Please observe the notes on copyright and usage.

boundaries of legally regulated medical and therapeutic practices. The fact that a book containing action proposals is freely available for sale does not imply that its application with clients or patients is permitted for everyone.

Hypnosis 1

… … You've been dealing with an eating disorder for a long time … … But you've also felt for a long time, and now you're even certain, that it's not really about food … … Bulimia … … the act of devouring large, extremely large amounts of food and then vomiting it all back up … … It might seem contradictory at first, to eat as much as possible and then purge it all … … But it's not really contradictory at all; it's simply a reflection of your emotions, your feelings … … and in emotions, there's not just black and white … … There are conflicting feelings and tendencies … … like the desire for comfort and love, the desire for attention and recognition … … the need to fill up what's missing … … and at the same time, the urge not to be overwhelmed, not to be flooded … … and maybe even the feeling that by consuming so much food, you've made a mistake and now need to correct it … … and surely, you've had to correct things in your life many times … … steer against the tide … … fix something internally that you didn't want to be imposed on you … … or that you took on out of helplessness … … or out of fear ... ... Maybe this constant vomiting is a kind of resistance, an almost symbolic act ... ... maybe life has often felt sickening ... ...

... ... There could be many reasons for bulimia ... ... perhaps very specific ones that you know or suspect ... ... or maybe you can't quite explain the bulimia to yourself ... ... And you don't have to ... ... What's important now is to accept yourself, especially with the problems you have ... ... especially with bulimia ... ... because it is, or at least was, a part of your life, a part of your development ... ... Condemning it now would mean rejecting a part of yourself ... ... And that would lead once again to feelings of unworthiness or guilt ... ... But now is the time to be kind to yourself ... ... Life can be sickening sometimes ... ... who would know that better than you? ... ... Now, you can simply rest and use the relaxation of the trance ... ... You don't need to do much, just listen and let the words flow into your feelings ... ... Now, you can just be there for yourself and rest ... ... and then you'll find renewal and inner healing ... ... [20 seconds of silence] ... ...

+++ Variant 1: Bulimia, General +++

… … In the tranquility of trance, you are closer to your feelings than in a waking state … … You are now closer to yourself … … very close … … and in this closeness to yourself, you can make a pact with yourself … … a pact of change and inner healing … … healing of old wounds that once arose from disappointments and hurts … … from rejection and judgments … … judgments that others had or have about you … … also wounds from self-judgments that developed over time because you adopted external judgments and assessments … … It's time to end that … … Time to go your own way and leave all that behind … … So, you resolve and make a firm agreement with yourself to care for yourself attentively and lovingly … … You resolve to treat your body gently, to nourish it slowly and moderately, and to refrain from vomiting … … You will find better ways to get rid of what makes you feel sick … … much better ways … … absolutely … … [30 seconds of silence]

+++ End of Variant 1 +++

+++ Variant 2: Bulimia, Relapse +++

... ... In the tranquility of trance, you are closer to your feelings than in a waking state ... ... You are now closer to yourself ... ... very close ... ... and in this closeness to yourself, you can make a pact with yourself ... ... a pact of change and inner healing that you've achieved before, and that's why it will succeed now even better ... ... It will succeed now even better in healing old wounds that once arose from disappointments and hurts ... ... wounds from rejection and judgments ... ... judgments that others had or have about you ... ... also wounds from self-judgments that developed over time because you adopted external judgments and assessments ... ... It's time to end that again and for good ... ... Time to successfully walk your own path again and leave all that completely behind ... ... So, you resolve and make a firm agreement with yourself to once again and forever care for yourself attentively and lovingly ... ... You resolve to truly treat your body gently, to nourish it slowly and moderately, and to finally refrain from vomiting ... ... You will find better ways to get rid of what makes you feel sick ... ... much better ways ... ... absolutely ... ... [30 seconds of silence] ... ...

+++ End of Variant 2 +++

... ... Now, rest ... ... Just linger in your feeling and let the relaxation of your body become a deep inner relaxation ... ... You are close to yourself, and now you can rest and regain strength ... ... Here, there are no duties and no tasks to complete ... ... The time of bulimia is coming to an end and will become a life experience that will soon be just a memory ... ... It takes time, and you take that time ... ... You are recovering now and in your everyday life, because from now on, you will be more mindful of yourself and consciously and deliberately pay attention to your feelings and moods ... ... Now you feel good, and you feel freer and lighter every day ... ... more content and happier every day ... ... freer and lighter ... ... more content and happier ... ... every day ... ...

Hypnosis 2

Instructions for Conducting the Session

An anchor (or trigger) is a stimulus designed to produce a specific feeling or thought. It acts as a signal that the client perceives and that then initiates an internal process. The established anchor then replaces the suggestion. In everyday life, a client can use an anchor to initiate or create a desired state even without being in a trance state. Various stimuli can be used as anchors/triggers. I work with the following options, which I also use in the "Ten Hypnoses" series:

- Physical anchors (closing the hand, pressing the thumb pad ...)

- Visual anchors (symbols, word cards ...)

- Auditory anchors (sound signals like a phone ringing, melodies ...)

- Olfactory anchors (scented oils ...)

- Tactile anchors (pocket stones, talismans ...)

I also distinguish between peri-hypnotic and post-hypnotic anchors. Peri-hypnotic anchors are those used primarily during hypnosis, where the therapist sets up the anchor and then repeatedly triggers it as a supplement to the suggestions and visualizations. Post-hypnotic anchors are primarily set up for use after the session, so the client can help themselves with them. Have a card ready with the inscription "I am worth treating my feelings and my body with care and attention," and discuss with the client before the hypnosis that you will hand them the card during the session. They don't need to open their eyes for this. Simply announce the touch again shortly before passing the card and then touch the client's hand with it so they can grasp it. Just follow the instructions in the text!

+++ End of Instructions +++

...... Today, we will set up an anchor for you ...... An anchor is a simple tool that helps you shut down any impulse of bulimia as it arises ...... Whenever you feel the urge to eat hastily or experience a craving, you can use the anchor to quickly find inner calm and balance and choose not to eat

... ... Normally, an anchor holds a ship in place, ensuring it remains steady even in storms and high waves ... ... This is what your anchor will do for you, helping you stay grounded, stay centered ... ... especially when you feel those old bulimic impulses tugging at you ... ... And you should be able to carry your anchor with you ... ... at first, it will help you release the unwanted impulses ... ... to let go of the urge to eat hastily or excessively ... ... and then, as an anchor, it will ensure that you focus on inner balance, self-attention, and self-respect ... ... You have this important goal in mind, a thought that tells you ... ... I am worth treating my feelings and my body with care and attention ... ... You want to firmly anchor this thought so that you can truly feel free and healthy and move forward ... ...

[Have a card ready with the inscription "I am worth treating my feelings and my body with care and attention," and discuss with the client before the hypnosis that you will hand them the card during the session. They don't need to open their eyes for this. Simply announce the touch again shortly before passing the card and then touch the client's hand with it so they can grasp it. Just follow the instructions in the text!] ...

... ... But first, you need to relax and feel good, focus on the future ... ... right now, at this very moment ... ... This is very easy, and you're probably already feeling relaxed and free, after all, you are in trance and deeply relaxed ... ... and with relaxation, you automatically feel better ... ... Now you feel relaxation, and with it comes inner healing, healing of painful memories and difficult experiences ... ... Now you feel what true healing feels like and how helpful a conscious time of rest and introspection is for it ... ... Now you can focus on your future and imagine having a healthy and normal relationship with food ... ... eating with moderation and mindfulness, without rushing ... ... without vomiting ... ... Pay attention to your feelings, look inside yourself ... ... Feel yourself ... ... The more you can now focus on yourself, in this moment, just on the feeling of relaxation ... ... at this very moment ... ... the better you can now feel that inner healing is truly happening and that you are changing inside ... ... Now you don't have to worry about anything ... ... Now you don't have to accomplish anything ... ...

... ... Now, in deep relaxation, you can meet yourself openly, end the bulimia, and take care of yourself ... ... It's much easier now than ever before ... ... You take yourself seriously at this moment and rest ... ... The more clearly you can feel the relaxation now, the better you can also focus on self-care and self-respect in the future ... ... So feel the relaxation and accept yourself ... ... Now you succeed ... ... You can feel peace and freedom ... ... Now I give you the card in your hand ... ...

[Touch the client's hand and hand them the card. They can keep their eyes closed.]

... ... Feel the card in your hand ... ... You know what it says ... ... it says ... ... I am worth treating my feelings and my body with care and attention ... ... You think about this sentence, this attitude ... ... You feel that you are now feeling well ... ... and now you focus on yourself ... ... you resolve to treat yourself and your body with respect, with your health ... ... The card reminds you that you can feel good, just as you feel good now, because that is always and everywhere possible ... ... especially when stress and hectic arise, and old patterns or bulimic impulses resurface ... ... The card always helps you when you carry it with you ... ...

+++ Variant 1: Bulimia, General +++

… … When you carry the card with you, you feel as well as you do now, because it reminds you of how well you feel now … … your whole body remembers, your entire organism remembers your goal, because you want to make sure that you treat yourself with respect and care, because that is the foundation for healthy and balanced eating habits … … This means that you can shut down the impulses of bulimia, the urge to binge and purge, and this leads to deep inner processing of old pains … … Your subconscious does this for you … … This card in your hands is your anchor … … the anchor that keeps you grounded in your inner place of self-respect and leads to a constructive processing of old burdens deep within you … …

+++ End of Variant 1 +++

+++ Variant 2: Bulimia, Relapse +++

… … When you carry the card with you, you feel as well as you do now, because it reminds you of how well you feel now … … your whole body remembers, your entire organism remembers your goal, because you want to make sure that you treat yourself with respect and care, because that is the foundation for healthy and balanced eating habits … … This means that you can once again shut down the impulses of bulimia … … this time even better than the first time … … because you've done it before … … and what you've done once, you can do even better now … … Your subconscious helps you and accompanies you on your path to success … … on your final liberation from bulimia … … This card in your hands is your anchor … … the anchor that keeps you grounded in your inner place of self-respect and leads to a constructive processing of old burdens deep within you … …

+++ End of Variant 2 +++

… … You can carry the card with you every day … … and whenever you feel that old and disturbing impulses are resurfacing, you can take it in your hand and read what it says … … I am worth treating my feelings and my body with care and attention … … and immediately you feel deeper calm inside and even a sense of emotional balance and healing … … just as you do now … … exactly as you do now … … even when you hold the card in your hand or touch it without reading it, you feel the liberation and the positive energy clearly ... ... just like today, every day, just like today ... ...

Hypnosis 3

... ... You want to end bulimia, to process your emotions internally and give up the hasty, extreme eating and subsequent vomiting ... ... Deep in your thoughts, deep in your feelings, there is a land of infinite possibilities ... ... the land of dreams, which consists only of feelings, and it's here that you can change everything ... ... because in the land of dreams, you find your own creativity ... ... your creative thoughts and your creative solutions ... ... You enter the land of dreams ... ... You're already there, because a part of you is always there ... ... always deep in your feelings ... ... You take a deep breath in and out, and then you feel that you are there ... ... You look around

... ... You are standing in a blooming summer meadow ... ... the sun is shining, and it's pleasantly warm ... ... Your gaze goes upward, toward the sky ... ... There are small white clouds being driven by the wind, and suddenly it feels as though all disturbing thoughts and feelings, all painful and burdensome memories are being carried away by the white clouds ... ... In the land of dreams, this is possible ... ...

Here, the wind frees you from pain and problems … … and perhaps you think that such things are only possible in fantasy … … But fantasy and reality aren't far apart; they're actually very close to each other … … You think about the time of bulimia … … about the urge to gulp down as much food as possible, to stuff yourself, and then the subsequent vomiting because you regretted it … …

… … You walk through the meadow with your memories, but the memories don't hurt … … and deep inside, more memories surface, but nothing can harm you here, nothing can hurt you here … … because all the pain is being carried away by the clouds … … It's all just memory now … … Maybe you also feel sadness or tears inside … … Let them come, they're memories of your life … … Memories that can't hurt you … … You let go of the inner pain in the wind of the dreamland … … Maybe you know the reasons for bulimia, maybe you've recognized or understood much of what led to it … … and of course, there are always connections or backgrounds to our behaviors or problems that we don't understand … … yet you can free yourself from them … … The land of dreams helps you with that … … because that's what it's there for … … to help you … …

... ... Suddenly, you discover a well in the middle of this meadow ... ... You walk to the well and notice a sign attached to it ... ... The sign reads ... ... Well of Bulimia ... ... and it also includes an instruction, like a user manual ... ... It says ... ... Draw healing water from this well and cleanse yourself internally ... ... You wonder how this is supposed to work ... ... Next to the well, there is a bucket with a rope, so you can draw the healing water from the well, but how are you supposed to cleanse yourself internally? ... ... You look into the well, which is very, very deep ... ... With the rope, you lower the bucket into the deep well until you reach the healing water, then you draw up a bucket full of healing water ... ...

... ... Then suddenly, you notice that your entire body is covered in dust ... ... It covers your entire skin ... ... and then it becomes clear to you ... ... This is the dust of time, of memories ... ... especially the burdens and pains, all the memories and experiences that led to the eating disorder ... ... In the land of dreams, these experiences sit like dust on your skin ... ... Dust that you can wash off ... ... But weren't you supposed to cleanse yourself internally? ... ... Then it dawns on you ... ... You are in the land of dreams, and this is the land of your imagination and feelings … … So you are inside, and what you can seemingly wash off externally here is always an internal cleansing … … Is it that simple? … … Can you simply wash away old pains and burdens here? … … Yes, you can, because this is the land of dreams … … So you wash yourself with the water, and if you wish, draw more water to wash your skin … … Cleanse your inner self … … It happens in a magical way, freeing you from the eating disorder, freeing you from bulimia … …

+++ Variant 1: Bulimia, General +++

… … After you've washed away all the dirt and, with it, the entire bulimia, you continue walking through the meadow and come to a silver mirror standing in the middle of the meadow … … large enough for you to see yourself in it … … You walk very close to it and look into the mirror, which in the land of dreams always shows a reflection of your constructive future … … You see yourself in the mirror, as if in a movie … … You see yourself in your everyday life … … You see that you have returned to healthy eating habits; you've really made it … … You observe yourself eating … …

a normal portion … … and you eat slowly and with enjoyment … … no gulping, and certainly no vomiting … … and the best part is that you feel good inside because you sense that the old pains and old sadness, all that led to bulimia, have been resolved … … Your deep inner self has soon fully processed these causes and let them go … … The land of dreams is your inner self and does this for you … … [20 seconds of silence] … …

+++ End of Variant 1 +++

+++ Variant 2: Bulimia, Relapse +++

… … After you've washed away all the dirt and, with it, the entire remainder of bulimia, you continue walking through the meadow and come to a silver mirror standing in the middle of the meadow … … large enough for you to see yourself in it … … You walk very close to it and look into the mirror, which in the land of dreams always shows a reflection of your constructive future … … You see yourself in the mirror, as if in a movie … … You see yourself in your everyday life … … You see that you have once again returned to healthy eating habits … … You've made it once more, because you already knew the path to liberation ... ... This time, your cleansing goes deeper ... ... This time, it is more lasting ... ... Now you look forward to your daily life even more, because you know that you've become even freer now, and that's why it's much easier now to take care of yourself in the long term, to eat without gulping and without vomiting ... ... and the best part is that you feel good inside because you sense that the old pains and old sadness, all that led to bulimia, have now been completely resolved ... ... for good ... ... [20 seconds of silence] ... ...

+++ End of Variant 2 +++

... ... Then you continue walking ... ... step by step ... ... and you think about how this can become a reality, what you can so easily experience in your imagination here ... ... Then it becomes clear to you that it already is reality ... ... your inner reality ... ... because the land of dreams is deep inside you ... ... It has always been there ... ... I'm just telling you about it ... ...

Hypnosis 4

... ... Now let yourself fully sink into the comfort and confidence of deep relaxation ... ... because this is a true step of inner and outer liberation ... ...

... ... Now let yourself fully sink into the comfort and confidence of deep relaxation ... ... because this is a true step of inner and outer renewal ... ...

... ... Now let yourself fully sink into the comfort and confidence of deep relaxation ... ... and open your inner self to all these helpful words ... ...

... ... Now let yourself fully sink into the comfort and confidence of deep relaxation ... ... and let all the words find their way into your depth... ...

... ... You know it's time to take care of your health again ... ... and this thought is now truly significant ... ...

... ... You know it's time to take care of your health again ... ... and this thought reconciles you with the waning time of bulimia ... ...

... ... You know it's time to take care of your health again ... ... and this thought gives you the feeling of truly ending the time of bulimia ... ...

... ... You know it's time to take care of your health again ... ... and this thought gives you the secure feeling that now, at last, you can walk new paths ... ...

... ... You are now letting go of the eating disorder and building a healthy eating behavior ... ...

... ... Notice the relaxation of your body and recognize the special significance in it ... ... because body and inner feeling are directly connected ... ...

... ... Notice the relaxation of your body and recognize the special significance in it ... ... because body and feelings are always one ... ...

... ... Notice the relaxation of your body and recognize the special significance in it ... ... because as balanced as your body is now, so are you in your new feeling ... ...

... ... Notice the relaxation of your body and recognize the special significance in it ... ... because your new feeling lets you eat normal portions again, without vomiting ... ...

… … You are now letting go of the eating disorder and building a healthy eating behavior … …

… … In the depth of your feelings lie self-love and self-confidence … … and you can feel them again now … …

… … In the depth of your feelings lie self-love and self-confidence … … and you can make them even stronger and more intense … …

… … In the depth of your feelings lie self-love and self-confidence … … and you find these feelings even in dealing with food and eating … …

… … In the depth of your feelings lie self-love and self-confidence … … and these feelings help you today in your liberation and in your new beginning … …

… … You are now letting go of the eating disorder and building a healthy eating behavior … …

+++ Variant 1: Bulimia, General +++

… … You commit today and every day to healthy eating habits … … because this way, you repeatedly experience relaxation and calmness while eating … …

... ... You commit today and every day to healthy eating habits ... ... because this way, slow eating becomes your new and easy routine ... ...

... ... You commit today and every day to healthy eating habits ... ... because this way, you take control of your eating behavior again ... ...

... ... You commit today and every day to healthy eating habits ... ... because this way, you regain full control over your life, in every situation ... ...

... ... You are now letting go of the eating disorder and building a healthy eating behavior ... ...

+++ End of Variant 1 +++

+++ Variant 2: Bulimia, Relapse +++

... ... You are now repeating the liberation from bulimia that you have already successfully achieved ... ... because this way, you once again and permanently experience relaxation and calmness while eating ... ...

... ... You are now repeating the liberation from bulimia that you have already successfully achieved ... ... because this way, slow eating once again and permanently becomes your routine … …

… … You are now repeating the liberation from bulimia that you have already successfully achieved … … because this way, you once again and permanently take control of your eating behavior … …

… … You are now repeating the liberation from bulimia that you have already successfully achieved … … because this way, you regain full control over your life, in every situation … …

… … You are now letting go of the eating disorder and building a healthy eating behavior … …

+++ End of Variant 2 +++

… … Today, you have reached an important milestone on your path, and you reach an important milestone on your path every day … … because you have come closer to your goal, much closer, and perhaps even … … you have fully reached this goal today … … … … Today, you have reached an important milestone on your path, and you reach an important milestone on your path every day ... ... Every day, you reach an important milestone on your path to healthy eating, without vomiting ... ... and every day, you can reach your goal and be completely sure that you are treating yourself and your body with care and love ... ... What succeeds in your imagination here and today also succeeds in your feelings here and today ... ... and everything, absolutely everything, that succeeds in your feelings also succeeds in your waking life ... ... as surely as it does right now ... ...

Hypnosis 5

... ... You want to end bulimia once and for all ... ... Sometimes you've succeeded because there were phases when you could do without it, when you could resist the urge to binge and also resist the subsequent vomiting ... ... It's possible to end it and to build healthy eating habits again ... ... Actually, it's not really about the food; it's more self-punishing and destructive to force down so much and then spit it out ...

... [Note: I prefer to say ... vomit ... because that's exactly how those affected feel; you can decide for yourself. To a bulimic patient who was lying in a hospital bed after a car accident, I once said ... You felt like life had torn you to pieces, swallowed you down, and vomited you into this hospital bed. She replied that no one had ever described her situation more accurately. She ended her bulimia while still in the hospital bed] ...

... This is the path you take today ... ... Today, you build a new inner attitude that will help you from now on to always treat your feelings and your body with care and eat healthily ... ... with moderation and especially without vomiting ... ...

... ... On this path, mindfulness helps you most of all ... ... mindful care of yourself ... ... That sounds quite simple, and with the right approach, it is ... ... Many things we set out to do are easier than we think if we go about it the right way ... ... if we choose the best path to reach our goals ... ... You have chosen the path of trance, the path of hypnosis ... ... And that is a path of good and helpful suggestions ... ...

... ... If there were an especially good suggestion, a formula that could help you, without tricks and without any trance, to always take care of your body and your feelings, so that you can eat normally and healthily, absolutely without binging and absolutely without vomiting, then you would surely want to use this suggestion ... ... Such a formulation, such a formula, does indeed exist ... ... and we call this helpful formula an affirmation ... ...

... ... And today, you will hear a very special affirmation ... ... an affirmation that you can use yourself to always attune yourself to truly staying on your healthy path ... ... You can use this affirmation today, in just a few moments ... ... by hearing it and allowing it to unfold its helpful effect … … and by repeating it internally … … even and especially outside of trance … … Once your subconscious has accepted it, it unfolds its good effect ever further … …

… … So now listen to your good affirmation … … Hear it and recognize its value, and as soon as you are sure that this affirmation is exactly what is good for you, you allow your subconscious to accept it … … and who knows … … maybe you've already granted that permission so that it works even better and faster for you … {5-10 seconds pause} …

+++ Variant 1: Bulimia, General +++

… … I accept my feelings and my body with love, and with love, I care for healthy eating and give up vomiting … …

+++ End of Variant 1 +++

+++ Variant 2: Bulimia, Relapse +++

… … I know that I can love myself, and therefore, I am worth it to finally let go of bulimia … …

+++ End of Variant 2 +++

… … And now these words sink deep into your inner self, deep into your feelings … … The suggestion you've heard, your very special affirmation for self-love and healthy eating, may now, with your permission, work deep within you … … and take a firm place within you … … as a firm and stable belief … … as the foundation of your new emotionality … … for self-love and self-care … … for eating with enjoyment and moderation … … for a new and good feeling of life, entirely without bulimia … …

… … In simplicity lies effectiveness … … and in a simple attitude often lies the solution and liberation we seek … … You sought balance and recovery … … and with a simple and at the same time very strong attitude, you have found a good path to it … … and you find it again and again when you say …

+++ Variant 1: Bulimia, General +++

… … I accept my feelings and my body with love, and with love, I care for healthy eating and give up vomiting … …

+++ End of Variant 1 +++

+++ Variant 2: Bulimia, Relapse +++

… … I know that I can love myself, and therefore, I am worth it to finally let go of bulimia … …

+++ End of Variant 2 +++

… … Now let these words sink even deeper into your innermost being … … Allow these words to take a firm place within you … … a place of peace … … a place of healing … … a place of life … …

… … In trance, loving words and affirmations become inner attitudes when they serve your goal and your possibilities … … especially when they are carried by respect and devotion to yourself and are formulated accordingly … … Your goal is your liberation from bulimia, once and for all, and thus a return to self-respect and self-love … … and this goal is served by your affirmation … … that is why it has already become your conviction … …

… … And whenever you say your affirmation in a mindful moment, you strengthen and support your mindfulness in dealing with yourself and ensure lasting success … …

Hypnosis 6

… … While you can feel the contact of your body with the surface you're lying on and at the same time feel the contact of your head with the pillow if you pay attention to it, you also feel the ambient temperature and can assess whether it is rather mild, cool, or warm, and meanwhile, you hear my voice clearly and distinctly … … and you feel the desire to regain a healthy eating behavior … …

… … You can feel the blanket on your body and touch it with your hands, and of course, you also feel that it warms your body a bit while the music plays in the background … … as you increasingly reject the hasty gulping down of food, more clearly seeking and finding your liberation … …

… … My voice is clear and audible … … It's easy for you to follow my words and reflect on them … … And so you can also think critically about bulimia, reject it out of conviction, and focus on healthy eating habits again … …

+++ Variant 1: Bulimia, General +++

… … You can let every sound become clear if you focus on it, while deciding that sounds coming from outside should now recede into the background because they are unimportant, and you can more focus on the helpful words you hear, maybe because you are more interested in them, or you simply let everything flow as it happens … … and you end bulimia with the next breath … …

… … If the temperature in the room were to change significantly, you would probably notice it immediately, and surely you would also notice if my voice suddenly became louder or softer, and with a little attention, you would certainly feel any clear change … … Just as you now feel the sudden change in your attitude toward eating, and you feel that you want to eat with respect and moderation again … …

… … You feel your body, and you feel your surroundings. You can perceive the outer world as well as the inner world, the feelings … … and more and more, you realize that you have more pleasant feelings in your inner depth than you thought, and suddenly you discover a new feeling of self-love and self-respect, and you want to bring this respect to yourself, especially when eating … …

+++ End of Variant 1 +++

+++ Variant 2: Bulimia, Relapse +++

… … You can let every sound become clear if you focus on it, while deciding that sounds coming from outside should now recede into the background because they are unimportant, and you can more focus on the helpful words you hear, maybe because you are more interested in them, or you simply let everything flow as it happens … … and you repeat the end of bulimia, you already know how to do it … …

… … If the temperature in the room were to change significantly, you would probably notice it immediately, and surely you would also notice if my voice suddenly became louder or softer, and with a little attention, you would certainly feel any clear change … … Just as you now clearly reject bulimia, you feel that you want to eat with respect and moderation for all time … …

… … You feel your body, and you feel your surroundings. You can perceive the outer world as well as the inner world, the feelings … … and more and more, you realize that there is a wealth of pleasant feelings in your inner depth, and immediately you find self-love and self-respect, and you want to bring this respect to yourself, especially when eating ... ...

+++ End of Variant 2 +++

... ... You can now feel the relaxation of your body, this beautiful and pleasant trance, and with each breath, this relaxation can go further, can take you deeper and deeper, so deep that you feel as if you are sinking into yourself and thus reaching deeper and deeper into your inner world, the world of your feelings, and as soon as this state of relaxation has set in and you feel that you are already very deep in relaxation and thus deep in your feelings ... ... you also feel directly that you have ended bulimia, that you have found a new way of dealing with yourself, that you have found self-respect and self-love, and therefore, you shape your day with these feelings ... ... and you approach every meal with respect and moderation ... ... for your health and for your self-love ... ...

Hypnosis 7

... ... You have an important goal, one that you have decided for yourself and especially voluntarily ... ... You want to overcome the eating disorder and eat in moderation again, without vomiting ... ... You can reach this goal most quickly when you take a clear stance on it ... ... when you fully focus internally on a new attitude ... ... Now this is possible because you are in trance ... ... Now it is happening just as you will it ... ... Focus on the external and then turn your gaze inward ... ... It's very simple ... ... Just follow my voice, which guides you safely and successfully ... ...

... You feel the contact of your body with the surface you're lying on ... [about 5 seconds pause] ...

... You also feel the contact of your head with the pillow ... [about 5 seconds pause] ...

... You can feel the temperature of the surroundings ... [about 5 seconds pause] ...

... At the same time, you hear my voice clearly and distinctly ... [about 5 seconds pause] ...

... And you feel the desire for healthy eating habits ... [about 5 seconds pause] ...

... You can feel the blanket on your body ... [about 5 seconds pause] ...

... The blanket warms your body ... [about 5 seconds pause] ...

... And in the background, the music plays ... [about 5 seconds pause] ...

... And you reject the hasty gulping down of food ... [about 5 seconds pause] ...

... Because you seek and find liberation within yourself ... [about 5 seconds pause] ...

... My voice is really clear and audible ... [about 5 seconds pause] ...

... It's easy for you to follow my words and reflect on them ... [about 5 seconds pause] ...

... And you have a critical attitude towards bulimia ... [about 5 seconds pause] ...

... You increasingly reject bulimia ... [about 5 seconds pause] ...

... You prefer healthy eating habits, without vomiting ... [about 5 seconds pause] ...

+++ Variant 1: Bulimia, General +++

... You can make every sound clear ... [about 5 seconds pause] ...

... You can decide which sounds are important ... [about 5 seconds pause] ...

... And you can be interested in truly helpful words ... [about 5 seconds pause] ...

... At the same time, you can let your thoughts flow freely ... [about 5 seconds pause] ...

... Now you end bulimia ... Now ... [about 5 seconds pause] ...

... You would immediately notice any change in the room ... [about 5 seconds pause] ...

... You would notice if my voice suddenly became louder or softer ... [about 5 seconds pause]

... With some attention, you would surely feel any clear change ... [about 5 seconds pause] ...

... Likewise, you feel a new attitude towards eating within you ... [about 5 seconds pause] ...

... From now on, you want to eat with moderation and respect ... [about 5 seconds pause] ...

... You feel your body, and you feel your surroundings ... [about 5 seconds pause] ...

... You can perceive the outer and the inner, the feelings ... [about 5 seconds pause] ...

... You also feel in the inner, especially pleasant feelings ... [about 5 seconds pause] ...

... Feelings of self-love and self-respect ... [about 5 seconds pause] ...

... And these feelings will now accompany you at every meal ... [about 5 seconds pause] ...

+++ End of Variant 1 +++

+++ Variant 2: Bulimia, Relapse +++

... You can make every sound clear ... [about 5 seconds pause] ...

... You can decide which sounds are important ... [about 5 seconds pause] ...

... And you can be interested in truly helpful words ... [about 5 seconds pause] ...

... At the same time, you can let your thoughts flow freely ... [about 5 seconds pause] ...

... Now you repeat the end of bulimia ... Now for good ... [about 5 seconds pause] ...

... You would immediately notice any change in the room ... [about 5 seconds pause] ...

... You would notice if my voice suddenly became louder or softer ... [about 5 seconds pause]

... With some attention, you would surely feel any clear change ... [about 5 seconds pause] ...

... You especially feel the rejection of bulimia ... [about 5 seconds pause] ...

... You want to eat with moderation and respect for all time ... [about 5 seconds pause] ...

... You feel your body, and you feel your surroundings ... [about 5 seconds pause] ...

... You can perceive the outer and the inner, the feelings ... [about 5 seconds pause] ...

... You feel this abundance of pleasant feelings ... [about 5 seconds pause] ...

... Feelings of self-love and self-respect ... [about 5 seconds pause] ...

... And these feelings will accompany you forever at every meal ... [about 5 seconds pause] ...

+++ End of Variant 2 +++

... You can now feel the relaxation of your body even better ... [about 5 seconds pause] ... And with every breath, this relaxation can go further ... [about 5 seconds pause] ...

... And in this relaxation, you can feel yourself well ... [about 5 seconds pause] ... ... But above all, you feel the end of bulimia ... [about 5 seconds pause] ... ... And you feel a new way of dealing with yourself ... [about 5 seconds pause] ... ... Self-love, self-respect, and moderation, especially when eating ... [about 5 seconds pause] ...

Hypnosis 8

Instructions for Implementation

The following hypnosis texts are structured so that they can be used as "normal" hypnosis or as self-hypnosis training. If you want to teach your client how to do effective self-hypnosis at home with this hypnosis, then also read the sections {Only for Self-Hypnosis Training}, which you can omit if you prefer a regular hypnosis session in your practice. A self-hypnosis trigger is a signal (action, image, or perception) that initiates the state of trance. With its help, even an inexperienced client can continue to work with self-hypnosis at home. Of course, they can "only" work with simple suggestions that they can remember well and that we should prepare, or with simple visualizations. Triggered self-hypnosis is a very good tool to give the client a task to take home, continuing therapy in the time between sessions. Completely self-guided self-hypnosis, without a trigger, is also teachable but requires a lot of time and practice. Setting up the trigger is quite a simple task and certainly eases the client, to whom I would not want to burden with practicing self-guided self-hypnosis. Despite all skepticism, I claim here again that there is really no problem in teaching a client a simple trigger self-hypnosis. It is no more dangerous than meditation, autogenic training, or yoga. People also survive those unscathed at home. I have witnessed many patients in my practice who not only managed well with self-hypnosis but enjoyed it. And if a patient enjoys self-hypnosis, no matter how simple the suggestion in the main part may seem, it is a very good support for compliance.

+++ End of Instructions +++

… … Today, you can free yourself from blockages in your thoughts, from all thoughts that can slow you down or hold you back … … You already feel a pleasant relaxation … … and in a few moments, your relaxation will go even deeper … … and at the same time, your deep inner self, your subconscious, will learn how simple and quick it is to end disturbing thoughts … … to end the ifs and buts … … to end hesitation and wavering and be free … … You learn this in this hypnosis … … {Only for Self-Hypnosis Training: … You can even learn to do this hypnosis yourself, because that too is easy ... I'll show you how it works, and as if by itself, your subconscious will learn in today's hypnosis how you can quickly and reliably do self-hypnosis ... anytime and anywhere you want ...} ...

... ... You simply come into a deeper relaxation, in which it is also very easy to let go of disturbing thoughts, even blockages that you cannot grasp ... ... Imagine a red rose in front of a white background ... ... a red rose in front of a white background ... ... Look at this rose ... ... Look only at the red rose because that makes all thoughts fade, and you come to rest ... ... It's very simple ... ... Just imagine the red rose in front of a white background and wait for the deep calm that arises ... ... the deep and liberating calm that spreads within you ... ... Maybe you already feel how this calm is spreading ... ... Feel the calm and tiredness ... ... or maybe you are already so calm that you feel completely free ... ... {Only for Self-Hypnosis Training: ... Whenever you close your eyes to find deep and liberating calm and imagine the red rose in front of the white background, you immediately go into a pleasant and comfortable trance ... just like now ... simply close your eyes, breathe calmly, and then look at the red rose and stay with this image, with this idea, until you become tired ...} ...

... ... Today, you want to end the eating disorder, to end bulimia ... ... Maybe you have a specific reason for the extreme eating and subsequent vomiting ... ... perhaps you know why you do it ... ... or maybe you can't exactly say why and how it came about ... ... But in any case, you can free yourself and let go of disturbing thoughts, burdensome self-judgments, and outdated thought and behavior patterns to simply feel free ... ... to approach new experiences and decisions openly and freely ... ... But first, relax even deeper, then it is even easier to really become free ... ... Imagine you are walking down ten steps of relaxation into deep freedom ... ... and with each step, you say ... ... I relax once more deeply ... ... I relax twice more deeply ... ... I relax three times more deeply ... ... I relax four times more deeply ... ... I relax five times more deeply ... ... I relax six times more deeply ... ... I relax seven times more deeply ... ... I relax eight times more deeply ... ... I relax nine times more deeply ... ... I relax ten times more deeply ... ... and then you are very, very deep in inner calm ... ... Now ... ... {Only for Self-Hypnosis Training: ... That's exactly how you deepen your trance at home, in your self-hypnosis, simply by walking down the steps to deep freedom and counting as you've just heard ... and you will recognize and experience that you can relax deeply and talk to yourself at the same time ... You can whisper the words of relaxation and relax and keep full control ... very simple and very safe ...} ...

+++ Variant 1: Bulimia, General +++

... ... Now, in the pleasant relaxation ... ... in the depth of your thoughts and feelings, you can truly free yourself from bulimia, every day anew if you want ... ... End bulimia now by actively and consciously thinking ... ... I end today simply the binging and vomiting of meals ... ... I end today twice the binging and vomiting of meals ... ... I end today three times the binging and vomiting of meals ... ... I end today four times the binging and vomiting of meals ... ... I end today five times the binging and vomiting of meals ... ... I end today six times the binging and vomiting of meals ... ... I end today seven times the binging and vomiting of meals ... ... I end today eight times the binging and vomiting of meals ... ... I end today nine times the binging and vomiting of meals ... ... I end today ten times the binging and vomiting of meals ... ... And then bulimia is over ... ... You are free ... ... {Only for Self-Hypnosis Training: ... And when you put yourself into a trance and have deepened it, you can whisper this suggestion to yourself ... exactly as you heard it here and today, by whispering ten times ... ... I end today simply the binging and vomiting of meals ... ... twice ... ... and so on, until you say ... ... I end today ten times the binging and vomiting of meals ... That's how simple it is, and you can do it yourself ...} ... Now stay in this feeling of freedom ... ... Feel that you are completely free in your thoughts ... ... and can think what you want ... ... Feel that you have become free in your feelings ... ... Nothing can stop you ... ... because you have decided for yourself ... ... You are free ... ... You are truly free ... ... [About 20 seconds of silence] ...

+++ End of Variant 1 +++

+++ Variant 2: Bulimia, Relapse +++

... ... Now, in the pleasant relaxation ... ... in the depth of your thoughts and feelings, you can free yourself from bulimia once more, because you've done it before ... ... End bulimia now once and for all by actively and consciously thinking ... ... I have freed myself from bulimia before ... ... I have freed myself from bulimia twice before ... ... I have freed myself from bulimia three times before ... ... I have freed myself from bulimia four times before ... ... I have freed myself from bulimia five times before ... ... I have freed myself from bulimia six times before ... ... I have freed myself from bulimia seven times before ... ... I have freed myself from bulimia eight times before ... ... I have freed myself from bulimia nine times before ... ... I have freed myself from bulimia ten times before ... ... And then your body remembers, and bulimia is truly over ... ... You are free ... ... {Only for Self-Hypnosis Training: ... And when you put yourself into a trance and have deepened it, you can whisper this suggestion to yourself ... exactly as you heard it here and today, by whispering ten times ... ... I have freed myself from bulimia before ... ... twice ... ... and so on, until you say ... ... I have freed myself from bulimia ten times before ... ... That's how simple it is, and you can do it yourself ...} ... Now stay in this feeling of freedom ... ... Feel that you are completely free in your thoughts ... ... and can think what you want … … Feel that you have become free in your feelings … … Nothing can stop you … … because you have decided for yourself … … You are free … … You are truly free … … [About 20 seconds of silence] …

+++ End of Variant 2 +++

… …{Only for Self-Hypnosis Training} … … When you do self-hypnosis at home, proceed exactly as you experienced it here … … It's completely simple and safe … … Start with the image of the red rose and imagine it until you feel that you are calming down … … Then whisper the suggestion to yourself … … I relax once, twice, and so on, until you say: I relax ten times … … Then you whisper your special suggestion ten times … [Here, repeat the main suggestion again] … … Then you may rest, and to wake up, imagine you are standing in icy rain and then just say: I'm waking up – One – Two – Three … … Then you can open your eyes and be awake … … That's how simple it really is … … It works just like here and today … … You go into a trance, free yourself, and simply wake up again … …

Hypnosis 9

Instructions for Implementation

Ideomotor responses refer to the phenomenon where our body follows our feelings and thoughts with movements. In everyday life, this following is reflected in a person's posture, muscle tension, and movement patterns, which naturally change with mood and thoughts. In trance, ideomotor signals can be used to obtain information that the client cannot actively communicate. For example, the subconscious can answer questions with an agreed-upon finger signal. Of course, ideomotor responses can also be used suggestively, for example, with arm levitations and catalepsies. Ideomotor responses strengthen trust in hypnosis and in one's ability to change, thereby promoting therapy.

+++ End of Instructions +++

… … Today, you want to do something to return to healthy eating habits … … without the binging of large amounts of food and without vomiting … … and this works best in cooperation with your subconscious … … because in trance, in the beautiful deep relaxation that you now feel, you can truly work with your subconscious, and above all, your subconscious can and will confirm and prove to you that it helps you … … Your subconscious will confirm and prove to you that together you are successful and that you are truly calmer and more balanced from now on … … I'll show you how that works … … Perhaps you are already very curious about how it works, that your subconscious gives you a real sign … … one that you can recognize and verify … … You can experience that today; in just a few minutes, it's time … … So, let's go … …

… … Changes can always happen when we manage to build up and maintain a clear picture of our goal … … and this clear picture of the goal can then take effect … … it imprints itself so deeply that it becomes the next truth in our lives … … and you want to create the truth of mindfulness and health in dealing with your body, especially when it comes to eating … … So now it's about having a clear picture of your goal … … a clear picture of healthy eating habits, with moderation and slowness … … with small portions and enjoyment … … So imagine that and focus entirely on this idea ... ... Imagine watching yourself eating with pleasure, leisurely, without vomiting ... ... and stay concentrated on this mental image ... ...

... ... Stay entirely in this image now ... ... Imagine it as a photo or a still from a video ... ... and this exact image should shape your future ... ... because that's how it should be and stay ... ... that's how you want to treat yourself ... ... with self-awareness ... ... with self-respect ... ... with respect for your body and your feelings ... ... with respectful eating ... ... The more you succeed in maintaining this image and seeing it before your inner eye, the better your subconscious can make this image your next truth ... ... and as soon as your subconscious has accomplished this, and it will accomplish this, your right hand will close into a fist ... ... as a sign that you can really hold this inner image and it becomes the truth ... ... Your subconscious will show you when it is time, when it has taken this on for you ... ...

+++ Variant 1: Bulimia, General +++

... ... The longer you focus on the image of normal and respectful eating and self-respect, the more your right hand closes into a fist ... ... Step by step, your right hand closes into a fist, and as soon as it is closed, your goal has become the new truth in your life ... ... Your subconscious will do it; it will close your hand and tell you that from now on, you will eat with moderation and pleasure and will not vomit because that time is now over ... ... Your subconscious also shows you that the experiences and events that led to bulimia are carefully processed internally; therefore, you no longer need bulimia ... ... Your subconscious does not lie ... ... It keeps its promise ... ... Your hand closes into a fist ... ... and you have reached your goal ... ...

+++ End of Variant 1 +++

+++ Variant 2: Bulimia, Relapse +++

... ... The longer you focus on the image of normal and respectful eating and self-respect, the more your right hand closes into a fist ... ... Step by step, your right hand closes into a fist, and as soon as it is closed, your goal has become the new truth in your life ... ... Your subconscious will do it; it will close your hand and tell you that it uses the relapse into bulimia to process even more internally, to free you even more from the events and experiences of the past so that you can end bulimia once and for all this time … … for good … … Your subconscious shows you with the closing of your hand that the time has come to say goodbye to bulimia for good … … Your subconscious does not lie … … It keeps its promise … … Your hand closes into a fist … … and you have reached your goal … …

+++ End of Variant 2 +++

[Please try to be patient until the hand closes. Ideomotor signals are reliable signs, similar to kinesiology muscle tests. Here, we work with a mix of suggestive prompting and ideomotor communication. If you repeatedly say … Your hand closes into a fist … it has a suggestive effect, and the ideomotor response follows. By suggesting that good sleep is associated with this, a coupling occurs in the unconscious. The subconscious simultaneously confirms good sleep. If it couldn't produce good sleep, it wouldn't be meaningful to close the hand. So if the closing occurs only due to the suggestion, that's still proof of its effectiveness for the mind, since it was "agreed upon" that way. If the mind is convinced, the goal is almost achieved].

… … Your subconscious has anchored the image, and therefore, from now on, you will prefer healthy and balanced eating habits … … Your hand will now become fully mobile again, and you can open it … … Your subconscious hands you back full control of your hand, which may feel good … … You can check it … … Move your hand or both and your fingers and check that your hands are fully under your conscious control … …

[Always ensure that the client has regained full conscious and active control of their hands and fingers and can move them. Have them actively try. If it doesn't work, help with further suggestions … Your hands and fingers relax completely, they're very loose. Your hands and fingers are very, very loose … You can move them …]

… … Your subconscious has achieved your goal with you … … You helped with your mental image, and your subconscious helped by anchoring the image and with the feedback of the closed fist as proof that from now on, you will naturally focus on your goals and plans and achieve them daily and thus permanently … … Isn't it good that this proof is possible in trance? … … Yes, that's good … … That's really good because you know that today you were successful and that you will remain successful ... ...

Hypnosis 10

… … You know what it's like … to gulp down food in huge quantities and then vomit it all up … … You've experienced it yourself; it was like a compulsion, as if you couldn't do anything else, and maybe that's true … … You've tried to change that and somehow get out of it, to end bulimia and establish normal and healthy eating habits … … It hasn't worked out yet, but today is a new day … … and on every new day, you can achieve what is now on the agenda … … and today your goal is on the agenda … … Today you can end bulimia … … because today you're doing it differently than before … … It's much easier today because you just have to be inwardly ready for a real change … …

… … This is your day … … that's why you're here … … for a real change … … You know that every change arises deep within yourself, grows there, and unfolds … … It always goes from the inside out … … through self-respect and self-love to the end of bulimia … … This is your path … … This is your path of liberation … … This is your path of new beginnings … … You walk it with and in your thoughts and with and in your feelings … … … … You speak to yourself, to your deepest inner being … … You know who you are and what you can do … … So it's especially important that you say to yourself … …

… … I accept the fading time of bulimia as part of my life … … because I know that this is my path to inner peace … …

… … {about 5-10 seconds of silence} …

… … I accept the fading time of bulimia as part of my life … … because I know that every experience is an important part of me … …

… … {about 5-10 seconds of silence} …

… … I accept the fading time of bulimia as part of my life … … because I know that with self-respect, I can overcome any eating disorder … …

… … {about 5-10 seconds of silence} …

… … I accept the fading time of bulimia as part of my life … … because I know that hand in hand with myself, I can start anew … …

… … {about 5-10 seconds of silence} …

... ... I accept the fading time of bulimia as part of my life ... ... because I know that I am truly worth living in inner peace ... ... {about 5-10 seconds of silence} ...

+++ Variant 1: Bulimia, General +++

... ... I forgive myself for having harmed myself with bulimia ... ... because I realize that guilt feelings would only unnecessarily burden me ... ...

... ... {about 5-10 seconds of silence} ...

... ... I forgive myself for having harmed myself with bulimia ... ... because I realize that even the eating disorder contributed to my growth ... ...

... ... {about 5-10 seconds of silence} ...

... ... I forgive myself for having harmed myself with bulimia ... ... because I realize that there are no unnecessary experiences ... ...

... ... {about 5-10 seconds of silence} ...

... ... I forgive myself for having harmed myself with bulimia ... ... because I realize that all experiences shape me and make me stronger ... ...

... ... {about 5-10 seconds of silence} ...

... ... I forgive myself for having harmed myself with bulimia ... ... because I realize that by doing so, I am once again in harmony with myself ... ...

... ... {about 5-10 seconds of silence} ...

+++ End of Variant 1 +++

+++ Variant 2: Bulimia, Relapse +++

... ... I forgive myself for briefly relapsing into bulimia ... ... because I realize that guilt feelings would only unnecessarily burden me ... ...

... ... {about 5-10 seconds of silence} ...

... ... I forgive myself for briefly relapsing into bulimia ... ... because I realize that even the relapse contributed to my growth ... ...

... ... {about 5-10 seconds of silence} ...

... ... I forgive myself for briefly relapsing into bulimia ... ... because I realize that there are no unnecessary experiences ... ...

... ... {about 5-10 seconds of silence} ...

... ... I forgive myself for briefly relapsing into bulimia ... ... because I realize that all experiences shape me and make me stronger ... ...

... ... {about 5-10 seconds of silence} ...

... ... I forgive myself for briefly relapsing into bulimia ... ... because I realize that by doing so, I am once again in harmony with myself ... ...

... ... {about 5-10 seconds of silence} ...

+++ End of Variant 2 +++

... ... I now take loving care of myself ... ... with the deep confidence that I can truly meet myself with love ... ...

... ... {about 5-10 seconds of silence} ...

... ... I now take loving care of myself ... ... with the deep confidence that I can truly come closer to myself ... ...

… … {about 5-10 seconds of silence} …

… … I now take loving care of myself … … with the deep confidence that I will truly find myself … …

… … {about 5-10 seconds of silence} …

… … I now take loving care of myself … … with the deep confidence that self-love will free me from any eating disorder … …

… … {about 5-10 seconds of silence} …

… … I now take loving care of myself … … with the deep confidence that a new chapter of life is beginning … …

… … {about 5-10 seconds of silence} …

Distribution, publication, and copying in any form are prohibited and subject to damages.

All Titles in the Series

Volume 1: Smoking Cessation
Volume 2: Anxiety and Restlessness
Volume 3: Burnout
Volume 4: Reducing Overweight
Volume 5: Coping with the Past
Volume 6: Suicidal Thoughts and Attempts
Volume 7: Psycho-Oncology
Volume 8: Obsessions and Tics
Volume 9: Self-Confidence and Decision-Making
Volume 10: Grief Work
Volume 11: Psychosomatics
Volume 12: Chronic Pain
Volume 13: Depressive Thoughts
Volume 14: Panic Attacks
Volume 15: Domestic Violence, Victim Support
Volume 16: Post-Traumatic Stress
Volume 17: Exam Anxiety and Stage Fright
Volume 18: Anti-Violence Training, Offender Support
Volume 19: Addiction Tendencies
Volume 20: Social Phobia and Fear of Contact
Volume 21: Nail Biting
Volume 22: Self-Awareness and Self-Love
Volume 23: Teeth Grinding and Night Clenching
Volume 24: Feelings of Guilt
Volume 25: Fear in Crowds
Volume 26: Fear of Flying, Aviophobia
Volume 27: Fear in Enclosed Spaces, Claustrophobia
Volume 28: Tinnitus, Ear Noises
Volume 29: Fear of Heights
Volume 30: Neurodermatitis

Copying, publishing, and sharing with third parties are only permitted with the written consent of the author. Please observe the notes on copyright and usage.

Volume 31: Finding Inner Balance
Volume 32: Overcoming Loneliness
Volume 33: Fear of Illness, Hypochondria
Volume 34: Anticipatory Anxiety, Fear of Fear
Volume 35: Jealousy in Relationships
Volume 36: Driving Anxiety
Volume 37: New Start after Separation
Volume 38: Fear of Injections
Volume 39: Heart Anxiety Neurosis
Volume 40: Overcoming Resentment and Anger
Volume 41: Resolving Blockages and Positive Thinking
Volume 42: Stress Reduction, Stress Management
Volume 43: Body Relaxation
Volume 44: Deep Relaxation
Volume 45: Fear of the Dark
Volume 46: Falling Asleep and Staying Asleep
Volume 47: Compulsive Buying
Volume 48: Restless Legs Syndrome
Volume 49: Bulimia
Volume 50: Anorexia
Volume 51: Overcoming Nightmares
Volume 52: Imagined Deformity
Volume 53: Overcoming Distrust, Finding Trust
Volume 54: Processing Failures
Volume 55: Humiliation, Emotional Hurt
Volume 56: Distressing Compassion, Vicarious Suffering
Volume 57: Self-Forgiveness
Volume 58: Self-Awareness, Self-Confidence
Volume 59: Saying No
Volume 60: Assertiveness
Volume 61: Setting Boundaries and Self-Assertion
Volume 62: Decision-Making Ability

Volume 63: Success Orientation
Volume 64: Ruminating, Circular Thinking
Volume 65: Accepting Pregnancy
Volume 66: Birth Preparation
Volume 67: Spiritual Opening
Volume 68: Joy of Life and Inner Lightness
Volume 69: Patience and Inner Peace
Volume 70: Fibromyalgia and Rheumatism
Volume 71: Irritable Bowel Syndrome, Crohn's Disease
Volume 72: Fear of Nausea, Emetophobia
Volume 73: Stuttering and Cluttering, Speech Flow Disorders
Volume 74: Concentration and Knowledge Anchoring
Volume 75: Vitality and Spontaneity
Volume 76: Searching for Meaning and Finding Goals
Volume 77: Life Crises, Life Events
Volume 78: Workaholism, Goal Obsession
Volume 79: Helper Syndrome, Helpless Helpers
Volume 80: Medication Abuse
Volume 81: Gambling Addiction
Volume 82: Internet Addiction, Smartphone Addiction
Volume 83: Hoarding Disorder, Compulsive Collecting
Volume 84: Conspiracy Thoughts, Overvalued Ideas
Volume 85: Fear of Operations and Treatments
Volume 86: Fear of Aging
Volume 87: Travel Anxiety
Volume 88: Anxiety When Urinating, Paruresis
Volume 89: Fear of Intimacy and Togetherness
Volume 90: Fear of Blushing
Volume 91: Coming Out in Homosexuality
Volume 92: Charisma Training
Volume 93: Migraines and Chronic Headaches
Volume 94: Overcoming Allergies, Bronchial Asthma

Volume 95: Normalizing Blood Pressure
Volume 96: Compulsive Perfectionism
Volume 97: Sports Hypnosis, Motivation
Volume 98: Sports Hypnosis, Performance Enhancement
Volume 99: Determination and Focus
Volume 100: Encountering the Inner Child
Volume 101: Cravings, Binge Eating
Volume 102: Stimulating Metabolism
Volume 103: Bipolar Mood Swings
Volume 104: Borderline, Identity Crises
Volume 105: Hypomania, Euphoria, Mania
Volume 106: Restlessness, Agitation
Volume 107: Nervous Breakdown
Volume 108: Adjustment Disorders
Volume 109: Self-Alienation, Depersonalization
Volume 110: Ending Self-Pity
Volume 111: Primary Gain of Illness
Volume 112: Secondary Gain of Illness
Volume 113: Bullying, Victim Support
Volume 114: Letting Go of Envy and Jealousy
Volume 115: Fear of Spiders, Arachnophobia
Volume 116: Fear of Dogs or Cats
Volume 117: Fear of Strangers, Xenophobia
Volume 118: Excessive Worries, Generalized Anxiety
Volume 119: Strengthening Sense of Responsibility
Volume 120: Unrequited Love, Heartache
Volume 121: Work-Life Balance
Volume 122: Letting Go of Unattainable Goals
Volume 123: Allowing and Accepting Help
Volume 124: Letting Go of Adult Children
Volume 125: Tourette Syndrome
Volume 126: Life Changes and New Starts

Volume 127: Accepting Life in a Wheelchair
Volume 128: Understanding and Overcoming Homesickness
Volume 129: Understanding and Overcoming Wanderlust
Volume 130: Dizziness, Meniere's Disease
Volume 131: Overcoming Aggression
Volume 132: Cutting and Self-Harm
Volume 133: Hair Pulling, Trichotillomania
Volume 134: Postpartum Depression
Volume 135: For Relatives of Dementia Patients
Volume 136: Self-Harm, Artificial Disorders
Volume 137: Activating Self-Healing Powers
Volume 138: Preventing Depression Relapse
Volume 139: Reactive Psychoses, Follow-Up
Volume 140: Obsessive Thoughts and Impulses
Volume 141: Compulsive Checking
Volume 142: Compulsive Counting, Symmetry Obsession
Volume 143: Compulsive Washing, Cleanliness Obsession
Volume 144: Compulsive Questioning
Volume 145: Dissociative Paralysis
Volume 146: Phantom Pain
Volume 147: Overcoming Complaining
Volume 148: Hay Fever, Pollen Allergy
Volume 149: Sexual Abuse, Victim Support
Volume 150: Standing Strong Against Sexism, #metoo
Volume 151: Binge Eating
Volume 152: Overcoming Thoughts of Revenge
Volume 153: Detachment from the Aggressor, Stockholm Syndrome
Volume 154: Courage to Separate
Volume 155: Chronic Fatigue, Exhaustion
Volume 156: Fear of the Future, Existential Anxiety
Volume 157: Excessive Worry About Children
Volume 158: Fear of Failure

Volume 159: Ending Distrust and Control
Volume 160: Dejection, Dysphoria
Volume 161: Boreout, Chronic Boredom
Volume 162: Bipolar Disorders, Relapse Prevention
Volume 163: Mania, Relapse Prevention
Volume 164: Nihilism, Feelings of Worthlessness
Volume 165: Thumb Sucking
Volume 166: Being Brave
Volume 167: Being Proud
Volume 168: Overcoming Shyness
Volume 169: Being Able to Delegate Responsibility
Volume 170: Being Able to Show Emotions
Volume 171: Letting Go of Guilt, Victim Support
Volume 172: Processing Guilt, Offender Support
Volume 173: Mood Swings, Cyclothymia
Volume 174: Lack of Drive, Vital Sadness
Volume 175: Hearing Voices with Reality Reference
Volume 176: Confident Communication
Volume 177: Standing Up for Oneself
Volume 178: Taking New Paths
Volume 179: Confident Job Application
Volume 180: No Longer Being Taken Advantage Of
Volume 181: End of Submissiveness
Volume 182: Depressive Numbness
Volume 183: Mood Drops, Affective Incontinence
Volume 184: Mood Instability
Volume 185: Somatoform Disorders
Volume 186: Stomach Ulcer, Psychosomatic
Volume 187: Accepting Amputation
Volume 188: Overcoming and Letting Go of Hatred
Volume 189: Ending Accusations
Volume 190: Allowing Tears, Being Able to Cry

Volume 191: Finding and Sorting Repressed Feelings
Volume 192: Somatoform Pain
Volume 193: Living Autonomously
Volume 194: Anhedonia, Joylessness
Volume 195: Persistent Sadness
Volume 196: Obesity, Food Addiction
Volume 197: Parents of Abused Children
Volume 198: Letting Go and Letting Be
Volume 199: Childhood Sexual Abuse
Volume 200: Fear of Loss

www.ingramcontent.com/pod-product-compliance
Lightning Source LLC
Chambersburg PA
CBHW030452220526
45464CB00006B/2507